Love in an Emotional Support Group

Introduction

Emily McMillan is an incredibly talented romance novelist who owns a lovely boutique and is committed to critical environmental causes and loves writing about heartfelt romance and feel-good nostalgia.

Love in an Emotional Support Group is for those who love sharing the fog rolling in on a beach, redwood trees with lush ferns at the base, and bright wildflowers with someone you are in love with.

This novel is about two young professors who form an emotional support group and while leading this eclectic community find themselves attracted to each other. They spend time on lonely beaches and in lush redwood forests as part of their courtship. They are gratified they have helped so many in the college community find happiness in whatever situation they are in, which draws them even closer together. The book follows their romantic life until the moment he gently slid an engagement ring onto her finger.

Love in an Emotional Support Group

The Beginning

Wright College is a progressive liberal arts college with a student body of about 700 students that is tucked into a small valley in the town of Winchester. Most of the 12 buildings are constructed of red brick with ivy attached to the walls which gives it a charming look. The college prides itself on prompting students to develop strong character, academic excellence, and social awareness.

Heather Wellington, the director of student activities at Wright College, was excited about planning the student activities for the year. She organized parties, plays, musical performances for the students.

Heather planned many activities that prompted deeper thinking, were life changing, and would meet the emotional needs of students, staff, college leaders, professors, and members of the community. These included emotional support, self-awareness, self care, interpersonal relationship development, and career planning groups.

The intent was to challenge participants to protect themselves both physically, mentally, and emotionally. She understood that it was essential and was surprised to learn that so few in the college community recognized the need to bolster their emotional life.   Many did not know who to talk to or where to go when they were depressed so they just suffered in their damaged emotional state.

 Many turned to alcohol, drugs, and illicit sex, or just hid in a closet for hours at a time. She had seen so many within the university exhaust themselves and perform so much work that it affected their health and emotional state.

She recognized so many emotional problems on campus that did not require the assistance of a doctor, psychologist, or counselor and did not require medication to treat them.

She wrote children's, feel-good, nostalgia, love, and acceptance by others books which inspired her to meet the needs of the students. These reflected her sincere belief that everyone can have a wonderful and fulfilling life. Her writing described her love of natural settings such as foggy beaches, redwood forests with lush ferns, and pristine streams filled with little trout.

She focused much of her free time on environmental protection including preservation of endangered animal species and setting aside wilderness areas for all to enjoy their resplendent beauty and calming surroundings.

She spent much of her personal time advocating for equal

employment opportunity and was committed to cleaning the environment, providing financial security, and furnishing fair treatment for those who are marginalized, disenfranchised, and had been left behind.

Some just needed a few friends that they could share their lives with and discuss even the most weird, terrifying, and embarrassing situations they faced. There were introverts who had rarely had any friends and had no idea of how to reach out to their fellow students.

She felt that peer support was often sufficient to treat emotional problems and that some people were intimidated by mental health professionals, so they preferred to be treated by just ordinary people. Some felt jealous of the doctors because they knew they would never enter a highly paid profession with a lot of status. Some were afraid of the stigma associated with being counseled by a mental health professional.

Many students just needed the sense of community that is naturally developed among a group of academics who spend a lot of time together and are making themselves vulnerable to each other.

Many of the emotional problems she saw on campus were a product of difficult relationships. A lot of them stemmed from dating difficulties where either the boy or the girl or both were saddened by poor communications, insensitivity, or an unexpected breakup. Many were so much in love that they could barely function after the other person left.

The incoming freshmen were only 18 and may have never had a girlfriend or boyfriend, had not even gone out on a date, or had never kissed someone. They had not developed the ability to protect themselves emotionally if the relationship soured, and were particularly vulnerable to the sadness that a breakup can cause.

Some students were already overwhelmed with living outside the security of their parents' home, facing rigorous competition for good grades, having to share a room with someone they did not know or like, and being exposed to different lifestyles than they were familiar with.

Some who were very close to their family missed them so much they were physically weakened. She questioned whether an 18-year-old child should travel across the country just to attend a certain college, when they may just return to their hometown as soon as they graduate.

Some promised long-time girlfriends and boyfriends they would stay together when they both knew they would not. They felt guilty leaving that boyfriend or girlfriend behind when they could have attended a college or university close to home which would have provided the same quality of education.

Some were afraid of everything and were so anxious they could not sleep, eat, or carry on a lucid conversation. They just hid in their room until everyone left the house, so they did not have to interact with anybody.

She knew there was a great need for emotional support at the college, so she hurriedly sent an email to all professors, students, administrators, staff, and local residents about the chance to lead or participate in the emotional support group. Two individuals, Professor Eric and Professor Susan, volunteered to co-lead the group. Ten people who wanted to understand their emotions and heal from emotional problems and scars quickly joined.

The Co - Leaders

Professor Eric

Eric, a co-leader of the emotional support group, was a sensitive young man who cried at weddings, bar-mitzvahs, religious services, funerals, sappy movies, and celebration of life ceremonies. He loved to hug and be hugged for no reason at all and to cry when he felt like crying.

In stark contrast his father was a man of his generation. He owned a small factory which he ran until he was in his mid-nineties. He was rigid, harsh, unemotional, intolerant of mistakes, and criticized employees for any lack of skill or mistakes they made.

He was against charity because he felt poor people were just lazy.

He worked seventy hours per week, and he required his eight employees to work an excessive amount of overtime. He did not provide any benefits, paid vacation, or sick leave. The only paid time off they got was Christmas, New Years Day, Labor Day, Memorial Day, and the Fourth of July. The factory was sweltering in the summer, freezing in the winter, always dirty, and very dangerous to work in. He paid just two dollars per hour over the minimum wage which required the employees to work a second and third job to survive. His eight employees detested him but they needed the job so they suffered in silence.

He never told Eric he loved him or was proud of him. He

never took him fishing so he could feel the tug of a little bluegill flitting about the pond, and feel a sense of wonderment after catching his first fish. One of the saddest situations is a father who has never taken his son fishing.

Eric only saw him on Sundays and he was so tired from his self imposed grueling work week that he spent most of the day sleeping. Eric loved him but resented him for squashing his creativity and free-spirit.

Eric accepted his father's tyrannical approach to life but knew he could not do so forever. He was aware that his friend's fathers were approachable, merciful, and compassionate which made it harder for Eric to cope with his father and his negativity.

His father would dismiss any idea he had or plan he would make on a biased whim without even thinking about how it would affect Eric. He wished his father would think even a few seconds before telling him what to do and what not to do.

When his father was at the factory Eric read books on natural surroundings, protection of the wilderness, pristine beaches, interpersonal relationships, and small, cold streams with delicate rainbow trout darting from rock to rock.

Eric loved to hike and had a passion for wildflowers so he would stop hiking to focus on them for several minutes. When he was fond of a girl he would pick a little bouquet and hand it to her. She appreciated it because it was a more personal gesture than simply going to the florist and buying roses without much thought behind it. The young lady knew he was giving her something that was important to him. He loved all sorts of wildflowers, particularly the local ones that were blue and violet colored. Because he was so attracted to them he joined several native plant societies to be with like-minded naturalists.

His father told him he was misguided and wasting his

time on appreciating nature when he should have been working in his factory. His father searched his room when he was gone to ensure he was not involved with subversive organizations that placed humanity over order.

One day Eric realized he could no longer stand his father bullying him, and knew he had to leave.

He saw what his parent's marriage was like and he was disappointed in them for it. They could have had a much more pleasant life, and been better parents, but his father avoided emotional success for some reason unknown to Eric.

When his factory was not doing well financially he became surly and grouchy and wore grungy work clothes all of the time. He worked too hard and never developed any interests besides work.

He would stay up late paying bills or reviewing drawings the engineers gave him. He did not shave or comb his hair regularly and never ate with his wife.

Once she told him she was pregnant and he did not smile but just grunted and said you take care of it because I am too busy. It broke her heart that he called their baby "it"

Their marriage was a lifeless, loveless, distant relationship. She could not talk to him because he was so stoic, unemotional, and stubborn. Eric saw this marriage as a formal, legal entity only.

He wanted so much more for himself. He desired a girl he could sit by a campfire with and put his arm around her as they sat on a log just close enough to the firepit to feel the heat from the smoldering coals on a cool night. He wanted her to be fit so she could walk a mile or two with him in the early morning as the fog was lifting. She would excitedly point out a bunny rabbit on the neighbor's lawn as he hopped to the safety of his little hole in the ground.

She would love Eric and their future children and ensure they were safe, well-fed, and took their medicines and vitamins on time. She would dress stylishly in clothes that made her look cute to please him.   She would hire a carpenter to build a white picket fence surrounding their yard. She would plant a lush garden in front of the little house he bought for her. His wife would be content with what he could afford to give her and never push him to give her more.

His parent's life was not like that idealized vision that he had and he could not bear to watch their misery which greatly depressed him, so one day he walked to the kitchen and hugged his mother goodbye and

then stepped towards his father and said, "Dad I love you, but I gotta go." His father asked "Do you need money?" which was as close to showing affection as he ever did. Eric told him he had money and walked briskly toward the door. He hurriedly went to the bank and withdrew the $700 dollars in his account and closed it because he knew he was never coming back. He quickly walked three miles to the main road and stood with his thumb out until two men in an old rusted dirty blue truck stopped and said, "Where 'ya headed son?" to which Eric replied, "Anyplace but here." and the man chuckled and said "Hop in back." He stepped into the truck carefully to avoid the rust and leaned against the cab to avoid the wind that whisked by the truck.

The man dropped him off that night in a vacated downtown

with streets that were empty except for a brightly lit all night diner with about ten customers in it.

The diner reminded him of his favorite painting which was Nighthawks by Edward Hopper which depicted an all night diner in a darkened commercial district. It was the only lighted building in the area except the neon lighted bail bondsman down the block.

He stepped in and asked the ambivalent waitress for decaf coffee. She told him we have two kinds of coffee, caffeinated and caffeinated, and they are both bad.

It was an eclectic group that sat in the diner. There were a few overachievers wearing dark gray suits with power ties who had worked late into the night and needed a little boost before they began the long drive into the suburbs. A homeless man dropped his proceeds from panhandling on the counter and asked if she had any pie. She said "Which you want, honey, we got all kinda pies." The man told her apple so she brought him a large slice, warmed, with a dollop of whipped cream on top. He swallowed it like he had not eaten in days which was likely the case.

He had no idea of where to go but he asked the waitress where a nice park was and she replied "Sweetie, just follow that street for a mile." He thanked her, left the money on the table, and started to walk on the lonely,

dark, damp, creepy street. He
saw a few strange looking men
along the way but stepped away
from them and walked just a
little faster to get away from
them. He had hoped he could
just sleep in the park that night
and find a more suitable place
to live in the morning.

There were several homeless
people leaning against the
darkened brick buildings
shivering because they had but
a single blanket to keep them
warm on this chilly damp night.

Eric had never seen despondent people sleeping in the street before because in his town everyone had a job and a place to live.

He got to the park and curled up in the needles that had collected at the base of a large pine tree and fell asleep. He awoke to the sun shimmering between the needles and was well rested from his night's sleep outside. Eric was an Eagle Scout and had spent many enjoyable nights camping and backpacking and was always refreshed after a good night's sleep in the fresh air.

He started searching for apartments and saw an ad for a large, ultra-clean one bedroom apartment on 11th Street. He was not sure where that was so he asked a girl sitting on the freshly mowed grass with her legs crossed who was lost in a book on nature poetry by Susan Warner, where that was. She said "Good morning, it is close, just turn the corner and walk a half mile." He saw the manicured gardens in the park and told the girl how lovely he thought they were and she smiled and said I love them too. He nodded and thanked her and quickly walked in that direction.

As he walked he had a moment of panic and wondered what he had done. He had left home with very little clothing and a bottle of medication for anxiety which his father criticized him for taking because mental health medicine was for sissies. He had no family, no friends, and had no idea how to find a job. He started wandering the hilly streets of the city to prevent the boredom and loneliness he started to feel.

He was hungry so he found a little coffee house which was popular with the beat poets in the neighborhood. The coffee was not bad, but the croissants were stale and kinda crunchy. Customers hung out there for hours sharing their philosophies that had been developed during years of living at the edge of society.

He noticed what looked like a hundred specialized botany books and pictures of beautiful wildflowers on the wall which he looked at for an hour and then asked the owner, who had a PhD in botany, if he was a botanist. The owner retorted, "No, I majored in chemical engineering, but I sold all of the books when I graduated - botany is just a hobby."

Eric's belief and philosophy was that believing in Jesus was the only way to God and by knowing him your sins were forgiven and you will go to heaven. He knew that once he accepted Christ he was sealed by the Holy Spirit for salvation which he could never lose.

One customer had his three pound teacup poodle with him. Eric's family always bought large black labs so Eric was fascinated by the poodle and enjoyed watching it flit about while he sipped his now lukewarm coffee. A young English professor walked into the coffee house but Eric did not like him because He seemed egotistical and arrogant. He felt that proud people were self-absorbed and never considered anyone's needs or feelings but their own. The professor arrogantly walked to the counter and demanded that the owner serve him a large coffee with plenty of room for cream.

The owner served him and then the professor squeezed between two other people at the counter, poured his cream, and rushed out of the coffee house annoyed he had to be around riff-raff such as Eric.

A homeless man, who was carrying a half empty bottle of high alcohol content, artificially made wine, asked what he could get for the change he just placed on the counter. The change was not enough to buy anything in the store but the owner

gave him three fresh chocolate donuts and said "Thanks for coming in".

The owner was a kind gentleman who cared about his employees and gave them pats on the back and told them they were doing a great job, unlike Eric's father. He made sure they had plenty of breaks and could sit down and rest when they wanted to. He cooled and heated the kitchen so his employees would be comfortable even though his power bill was much higher because of his kindness.

An unkempt young man told Eric about a protest tomorrow to preserve a local wilderness area and asked him if he would like to protest with him. Eric said yes mainly to be around demonstrators with a social conscience and prevent his ever increasing sense of loneliness from getting worse.

The young man thanked Eric and said we will only have about forty people there so we need everyone we can get.

Eric arrived at the demonstration and listened to the passionate speaker talk about the natural beauty of redwood forests and how they were being cut down to use as construction materials.

After the demonstration ended Eric took a walk and started to think about his plans for life. He realized that he had no future, no formal education, and no job. He thought about what to do for a long time and eventually decided to go to college. He applied at Wright College and was accepted as a freshman which he was quite pleased about.

Because of his love for nature, he chose to major in botany. He found he was an excellent student and studied at the college for many years and eventually transferred to Warwick University to earn a PhD in botany. Shortly after he graduated Wright College offered him a position as a botany professor which he gladly accepted.

He was well liked because he spent time with his students on a one-to-one basis in addition to preparing engaging lectures. When he was not in the classroom he was performing research in the laboratory and in the field. He always wore grungy t-shirts with the name of the college on the front, and shorts. He wore tennis shoes rather than scandals so he did not injure himself when he walked through the dirt covered areas.

Professor Susan

Susan was a pretty fresh-faced sociology professor who earned her PhD just one year ago. Her hope was to help the community she grew up in to overcome poverty and unemployment. She actually grew up in a quite wealthy family. Her father was a civil rights attorney and her mother was an actress who performed throughout the state.

She lived on the affluent side of the tracks, but just a half-mile from her home, poverty was rampant. The residents of the neighborhood would listen to live music and dance in the street to forget their troubles for a moment but when the music stopped they were still poor.

Many suffered from malnutrition and had few, if any, teeth. Many had not seen a doctor in years because they had no health insurance and no money to pay a doctor so their health suffered greatly. They ate rice and beans almost every day and occasionally would find food in the dumpster behind the town's grocery store to break the monotony of their simple diet.

Susan always wore dresses and skirts which was unusual because most of the girls she knew wore Levis, but she liked being a girl. She had long blond hair which she kept in a ponytail to keep it out of her eyes and because she thought she looked cute wearing one. She had deep blue eyes and wore a teal headband to highlight them. She always wore a multi-colored hat outside so her light skin would not be darkened or shriveled. She walked softly, almost tentatively, without making any noise.

She tastefully decorated her tiny office with an antique table, a blue velvet covered loveseat made with hand carved wood, and pieces of lace throughout the little room. The hardwood floor was nice but she had to re-do almost everything else when she moved in. She brought in several plants which she would water daily and trim every week or so. She had a lot of pillows carefully placed throughout the office which gave the room a comfortable feeling.

Her decor set her apart from the other professor's offices which were stark and plain. The walls were off-white, dirty, and had cobwebs hanging from them. Aside from a diploma, a whiteboard, and maybe a 20 year old protest sign, the walls were usually empty. There were no plants and a minimum of furniture.

They only had one chair because they did not want anyone to linger in their office.

Susan would work so intensely that she would forget to eat and became quite thin. Her mother would chastise her for that when she visited them and made her drink protein shakes to be healthy and gain a little weight.

She wrote about social injustice and how society pollutes neighborhoods occupied by the poor and the disenfranchised. She was quiet but was still an activist. She wrote several books on sociology which included chapters on environmental justice which is the premise that poor people deserve as clean an environment as the rich have.

An outgrowth of that premise is if we provide a clean environment for the poor we should also provide financial security for them.

She often thought about the living conditions of those in her town who lived on the other side of the tracks and breathed polluted air and drank water tainted with lead and other dangerous contaminants, and vowed to improve their lives.

Organizing the Emotional Support Group

Professor Eric and Professor Susan met in her office to make plans for the emotional support group. He noticed how pretty she was which drew his attention away from planning the group. He noticed the plush interior of her office which he really liked a lot. She thought he was kinda cute which also distracted her from their planning work.

She flirted with him just a little bit. They both smiled at each other when their eyes met. He noticed her bright dress and stylish shoes which were pleasantly different from the running shoes that most of the other professors wore. He found her light hearted sense of humor refreshing. Susan could tell that Eric was passionate about emotional support which made him more attractive to her.

While still distracted by each other, they planned the group to meet for one year and attendance would be mandatory so the members of the group could develop a sense of community.

They decided to hold the gatherings on the first

Wednesday of every month from 9:00 am - 1:00 pm which they could do because members of the academic community had very flexible schedules.

Students were expected to be excused from class for the meetings and professors were expected to find a substitute to teach their class.

They chose a weekday because many professors and

students were so exhausted from the work week that they just needed to be at home alone to recuperate on weekends.

They both agreed that four hours was a long time so they decided to break the meeting up by hiring two speakers for each day, enjoying a continental breakfast, serving a hot lunch, and having hot chocolate and herbal tea available all day, and holding multiple discussion sessions, time for personal reflection, free time, and opportunities to share about a book they were reading or an artistic showing that was meaningful to them.

The speakers would be invited to talk about any subject that related to self-awareness, self-care, and emotional support.

They could share religious views, but only to prompt

members to think about how personal God is, but not to convert anyone. Talks on social welfare such as environmental justice, sustainability, green living, interpersonal relationships, and how to love themselves were welcome. The speakers were expected to encourage participants to share at a deeper level with those around them than they normally would.

What was said at the group was confidential except if someone was going to hurt someone or themselves and if someone needed psychiatric care. The group was to be a safe place where everyone would feel supported. Advice could only be offered in a spirit of peace and love.

Participants were encouraged to share their deepest thoughts, most miserable experiences, and utter failings, no matter how shocking and disgusting they were. Love for each other was to be unconditional.

Eric and Susan discussed beautiful locations to gather in and decided each meeting would be held in an aesthetic outdoor setting. If it was raining they could wear parkas with hoods and enjoy listening to each other while under umbrellas or portable awnings. Susan loved the rain and snow and envisioned herself cuddling up with Eric to keep warm on a cold, snowy, foggy morning.

Being part of the beauty and freshness of the cleansing rain compensated for the minor inconvenience it presented.

The group would be encouraged to build a fire to keep warm on cold and snowy days. Many found meeting with intimate friends while watching the snowflakes float to the ground to be a totally spiritual experience which served to make them consider a loving God and to love each other as a reflection of His love for them.

They chose beaches, forests, a quaint farm, a meadow, a large lake, a small pond, and a rockscape to meet in. While they were talking Susan thought about sitting around a campfire in a snowy meadow close to Eric, which made her more excited about the emotional support group.

For their first meeting they selected a beach that was empty during the week, and was known for its unspoiled beauty. They hired two speakers, one a psychologist who focused on interpersonal relationships and spirituality; and the other a philosopher who contemplated the resilience of the human spirit.

They arranged for a local upscale bakery to deliver croissants with strawberry jam, grapefruit juice, bacon quiche, and fresh fruit to the beach at 9 am.

They did not order coffee because Professor Eric and Professor Susan wanted participants to be calm rather than stimulated by caffeine.

They selected lasagne, organic salad, rye muffins, and sparkling flavored water for lunch at noon.

Then they sent an email to the ten participants announcing the first meeting and then Eric left her plush office with a slight smile, and she smiled back.

The Ten Participants

Stan and Alison

During the meetings Eric and Susan encouraged a young couple in the group who were freshmen at the college who said they were considering getting engaged and married and then spending the rest of their lives together, but were

terrified at the prospect of
that.

Both came from broken
homes and could see the pain
their parents experienced as
their marriage eroded away,
and ended in loveless
divorces.

Stan's parents were congenial
and agreed to shared custody
of the children and split their
assets evenly, but did not
shed a tear as they walked

out of their attorney's well decorated but cold office.

They still spoke, but only about business matters or the children, and each strained to say hello when they started the conversation, but it was difficult for both of them to do.

Stan never got over the divorce and it clouded every relationship he had with a girl.

Alison's parents spent three years in a contentious battle over custody of the children, their house, sentimental items, and assets. They spent over seventy thousand dollars on attorneys fees, just to get divorced. They avoided each other for three years while their marriage disintegrated and have not spoken to each other since. When absolutely necessary to communicate they did it through attorneys. Alison did not know whether she could trust either parent and was angry at both of them.

Eric reminded them that most first marriages do not end in divorce and are generally pleasant and loving as long as the boy and girl are compatible. The foundation of a marriage is for both the boy and the girl to have a growing belief in God.

He suggested that before getting engaged they talk about their goals, personalities, fears, mental and physical health, medications they take, financial status, debts, careers, plans to open a business, and desire to have children. Eric went on to say that the desire to have children or not was a critical issue and should be discussed well before considering engagement.

The group was excited for the young couple and could see that they were very much in love and that would carry them through the little squabbles they would have from time to time. Stan said he was committed to never yelling at Alison and always being kind to her. She replied she would be supportive, encouraging, and gently tell him when he was going to do something stupid.

As Eric instructed the young couple on the basic tenets of marriage he thought about getting married some day to someone like Susan. She pondered what Eric would be like as a husband and wanted to explore that side of him.

Helen

One of the members was a divorced woman in her thirties whose husband left her with a simple "I am leaving-goodbye" and walked out the door with a small suitcase. She shed a lot of tears as he walked out and became sad at the prospect of living the next 50 years without the love of her life. Two days later he sent a moving company to the house to pick up his clothing, and a few pieces of furniture, which she felt was unnecessarily insensitive. She was sad and needed to be with those who liked her and accepted her.

She was clinically depressed, was on three mental health medications, and spoke to a therapist at least three times per week.

Some members of the group suggested she throw her life into helping others such as those who have been divorced one or more times, struggled with their children, or also felt they needed therapy and medications. She went on to say she had been financially supported by her husband for the last ten years and had rarely worked before that.

She had no way to support herself and was running out of savings. Eric suggested she attend a university which would be free because she had little resources. She said she had always thought about going to college and would decide what she would like to major in soon. She was more optimistic at that moment than at any time since her divorce.

Helen confided that she had always wanted to be an artist or musician but was reluctant to because they usually led fragmented lives with an irregular income but her friends told her to follow her passion.

She was a talented and creative oil painter and planned to open an art school for children and would start advertising the business tomorrow. She was so excited and could barely wait to rent a studio. She had seen a small space in a nice shopping mall that she would look at tomorrow. The group applauded and entered into her happiness.

She said she could afford to pay the rent for a few months until she found some students. As she walked out of the gathering she had a glimmer of hope in her deep green eyes.

She had dated a little since the divorce but just did not really enjoy the guys she went out with. There were no single guys she knew and had tried online dating but found it risky, and never found anyone she wanted to go out with, so she canceled her subscription to the dating service and wrote a bad review about them.

She was frustrated that it was so hard to meet guys to hang

out with. Some were biased against her because she was divorced which frustrated her because it was not of her choosing.

Susan suggested she attend a divorce care group. She knew of several in the area and promised to send her information about them later that day.

Eric suggested going to a singles group at a church in town where she could meet someone her own age.She eventually joined a 20s and 30s singles group that was established for members to find companionship and a relationship that would eventually lead to marriage.

She met a handsome young man with a bright future there and within five months they were married.

During these discussions about marriage Eric's mind would drift to thoughts of Susan and how she would be a loving wife.

After two or three months Eric started to sit close to Susan throughout the meeting. She was demure and would wait for him to walk over to her. When it was cold he would sit close to her to keep her warm. During one cold morning while sitting on a log in the forest he took off his jacket and placed it around her slender shoulders. She said "You must be cold", so she stepped away for a moment and returned with a wool blanket which she placed on his lap and hers. It was so natural to lean against each other while they sat there on the small log under Susan's blanket. Eric wondered if she brought the blanket just for him, which she did.

It was time for a discussion session so they both slowly stood up from the log and stepped over to the campfire where the remainder of the group was sitting. Susan put the blanket away but kept Eric's jacket wrapped around her shoulders for the rest of the meeting.

Richard

Richard was a chemistry professor in his seventies who had just lost his wife and went on to describe their fairy tale marriage. They met at a youth group when they were sixteen and dated until they were eighteen and then immediately got married. They had been infatuated with each other since then. Their temperaments matched and each was careful not to control or manipulated the other.

They never yelled at each other and resolved any disagreement before retiring for the evening. He said he could not describe how much he loved her and was very sad that she died, but thankful for the decades they had together. They enjoyed every minute of raising their two sons together and were always proud of what good kids they turned out to be. He seemed able to take care of himself even though he was alone, but he had a home health care nurse visit once a week to make sure he was taking his pills and was in overall good health. He was not very good at cleaning so he had a maid come in every two weeks to tidy up. He hired a lawn service so the lush gardens in the front yard looked crisp, cool and moist.

John and Penny

John and Penny were in their fifties and worked in the human resources department at the college. They had a great marriage which sustained them through the ordeals of raising eight children. Only half of them could sit at the table at a time so they ate in shifts. Six of them were their own and two were her sister's who had lost herself in a world of foolish living and was in no position to raise them. Most of the time they did not know where she was. She could have been homeless, living in a sleazy, dirty motel, renting a broken down dirty trailer, staying in a skid row hotel across from the bus station, in a psych ward, or in jail.

The children did not understand why they could

not live with their mom. John and Penny could not tell them that their mother was totally irresponsible so they just made up excuses. The children pretended to believe the excuses but knew they were not true.

The eight children never felt deprived because John and Penny were always available to look at a good report card or a picture that they had drawn and give the child their

full attention. They were
happy and said they would
not change any part of their
life.

Eric and Susan really never
thought about having children
but over time she started to
secretly think about the
attention and care she would
get through her pregnancy
and the happiness of taking a
baby home to brighten their
lives.

She was sure their sons
would be handsome and their
daughters pretty and they
would both be very intelligent.

Larry

Larry was a third year
freshman at the college. He
did show up every meeting
but he looked like he had

slept in his clothes which he may have. They did not know where he lived or if he even had a home.

He was not a bad guy but he had no plans for his life. He worked from time to time but had no real friends, except those in the emotional support group.

They encouraged him to establish a career and have some plan for his life. They suggested he pick a major but he never really did. Each week they gave him a few names to call about a job and he usually contacted them. He would get hired but only worked for a few weeks and they never knew whether he got fired or quit.

James

James was a civil engineer who had recently graduated and found a good position within a few days.

At his job he had very little interaction with others except for discussing projects and engineering concepts. He spent a lot of time on construction sites where he had very little opportunity to speak with anybody at all. He wanted to know those in his life at a deeper level and develop some meaningful friendships. He was depressed because he had no real friends and his relationships at work were superficial at best. He felt the need for emotional support because he was at a loss when he needed someone to talk to about a problem or weird situation in his life. He had immediately signed up for the emotional support group after reading the email about it that was sent by the activities director, and became one of the more active and verbal participants. He mentioned things in his life that he had not been able to tell people about for years. He was not sure if he wanted to be a civil engineer for an extended period of time so he spent many hours reading career development guides and interacting with job searchers on career development blogs.

Jimmy

Jimmy was a dedicated Baptist pastor at a church near the college and wanted to explore who he was and how to expand his faith. He worked too much and wanted to learn how to relax and develop hobbies that would distract him from his demanding job. He felt that this eclectic gathering of supportive people would encourage him to look out for his well being and ultimately become a more loving pastor.

Some of the relationships he had with other pastors and members of his church were excellent but he often looked for input from additional sources.

He wanted those he was close with to tell him what the best course of action was in any circumstance.

He wanted to be more comfortable chatting with those he met in any situation such as in a grocery store checkout line, on the walking path, and while cheering for his children at a sports event.

Emily McMillan, the author of this book, interjects, to say

that a good friend is Jewish,
and happily accepted Jesus
into his life.

Debby

Debby was an ecology
professor who shared about
wilderness and urban
ecosystems that she was
committed to preserving. She
was from a farming
community and realized that

each farm was its own little ecosystem and must be protected from interference.

She felt that each ecosystem could be defined and were as large as a portion of a state or as small as an individual house with a green roof and lush gardens.

Debby felt that each ecosystem had a boundary which should not be penetrated. She said that each natural setting they met in was its own ecosystem, and could absorb the members of the emotional support group and still be protected.

She loved redwood forests where hikers could become enthralled in the massive trees surrounded by lush ferns and bright blue and violet wildflowers. She had photographed many forests and brought the images to monthly group meetings to share her passion and describe what brought her joy. When doing this she told the group about the need to protect the irreplaceable redwood forest ecosystems.

Because she was so passionate about protecting these precious environments, she became involved with any organization that advocated for their protection. She spoke, wrote, taught, and demonstrated in an attempt to maintain the natural balance in each area.

She loved doing the work although she was exhausted by doing so, but could not say no to these requests to do more. She felt if she passed on performing a worthwhile task, the other environmentalists would say she was not really committed to her cause. She had great difficulty in saying she could not perform the additional tasks because she was exhausted and would get sick often because of that. She needed to realize there were many others who shared the same cause and they would do what she could not.

She wanted the group to teach her to say no gracefully and not be manipulated by other ecologists into doing more than she could.

She needed to not be manipulated by their frowns or them saying a tentative "I understand", when they really did not mean it.

Kathleen

Kathleen was a philosopher who spent many hours in coffee houses where artists, philosophers, sociologists, and psychologists hung out and discussed their views on life. Most of the customers there were off-beat and bohemian-like. There were no captains of the football team or head cheerleaders there but instead those who wrote poetry, majored in botany, advocated for the wilderness, and cleaned ocean beaches after oil spills.

Few would climb the sterile and cold corporate ladder or become high-profile attorneys who defended major companies who polluted the lands of the poor and helpless.

There were many highly literate patrons in these coffee houses who shared their philosophies of life with each other, and chided those who disagreed with their thoughts.

She enjoyed talking with her friends at the coffee house late into the night even though some of them were a little

weird and wore odd clothing.
She did not eat breakfast
because she was never
hungry in the morning, and
because she was so busy at
work she would only take a
few minutes during her lunch
hour to get a hot dog with
pickles and onions from the
pushcart by the entrance to
the building. As soon as her
9-5 ended she rushed to the
coffee house, which served
no healthy food, and talked to
her friends late into the night.

When she left she was too
tired to cook so she would
pick up fast food or just eat
potato chips, and then
collapse into bed. Because of
her terrible diet she felt weak
and sickly all of the time. She
confided that the only time
she felt liked and accepted
was when she was in the
coffee house. She needed
the attention and acceptance
desperately, and found herself

addicted to the dusty little establishment.

Members of the emotional support group told her they liked her and thought she was a nice person, and there were many others who loved her as well. They encouraged her to go to work activities at lunch or those held just after five o'clock. She could email friends at lunch rather than work through most of the hour. She took their advice and slowly developed friendships with people who were not part of the coffee house community. It was slow at first because she would only send one email each day and many did not respond or sent a brief hello and that was it. So she started taking a little more than an hour for lunch and sent out four emails a day and found that at least one would engage her in a meaningful conversation.

Once in a while someone would ask if she would like to go out for sushi and she gladly accepted.

She realized that those who conversed with her and invited her to dinner must have liked her. She found herself less addicted to spending hours each night at the coffee house and started spending a reasonable amount of time with her new friends. She decided to eat a small but nutritious breakfast and took at least 30 minutes for lunch to get a healthy sandwich or organic bowl of soup. She swore off fast food and would go home at night to warm up frozen, but tasty, organic vegetable dishes.

She found she had more energy and joined a hiking club, a gourmet society, and book discussion group to meet even more friends.

As Eric and Susan heard her story they realized they both appreciated each other for their healthy lifestyles and openness to friends and co-workers.

Roger

Roger was an environmentalist who had advocated for a fresh, clean, unpolluted environment for decades. He owned an urban forestry and arboriculture consulting firm and had a long list of enlightened clients.

He was also an amateur historic preservation architect who wondered why the owners directed the architect to design the house in the manner that he did.

Roger specialized in the preservation of aquatic life, particularly rainbow trout. He loved the sleek small fish and would go catch and release fly fishing every chance he got. He removed the barb on the hook so the fish were unhurt when he caught them, and he always examined the trout to determine whether it was healthy or not before he gently released it into the cold trickling stream and watched it dart away.

He had bad experiences with incompetent doctors when he was growing up so he would avoid seeing them even if he was sick. He had not been to a doctor in eight years and ignored symptoms of serious diseases.

Members of the group allowed him to share the negative experiences he had with insensitive and less than intelligent doctors. Several members of the emotional support group told him that their doctors were kind, personable, and good listeners. They were highly skilled and were able to treat their maladies or made appointments with other doctors for them. Roger agreed to go in for a physical and found that he had several conditions that could lead to serious illnesses if not treated. Over the next several months he visited four specialists who treated his illnesses. He was thankful to the emotional support group for saving him from what could have been dire circumstances.

Keith

Keith was an introvert who had a great deal of difficulty reaching out to others because it stressed him out. The group pointed out to him that being alone even in the midst of a crowd was not healthy. We were not designed to be hermits but to interact with others and enjoy their love, encouragement, and acceptance. They suggested ways he might communicate to others without being overly stressed. They told him that he should make friends with those who were also introverted so neither would feel overpowered. He should join organizations suitable for those who were more reserved such as garden clubs, chess societies, and social service volunteer organizations.

Over the next several months he made a few friends that were easy for him to spend time with. When he shared he spent time with a new friend each week the group applauded him. They said keep it up and before long he would have a full circle of close friends which would brighten his life.

Eric and Susan's Romance

While enjoying a cup of gourmet coffee at an upscale little coffee house they discussed how they felt closer to each other when they helped someone reach a level of emotional stability and learn to love others and love themselves.

Eric and Susan were gratified that they helped the members of the group to take care of their physical, emotional and spiritual needs. The year was over and they were happy that many of the group members became close friends.

Many times during the year they had lingered after the meetings and walked through a scented pine forest, or strolled on the wet sand on a pristine beach with waves crashing on the rocks at the shoreline. Because each had volunteered to lead the group they met and were able to develop such a wonderful relationship.

They were now very close to each other and would hike through the forest and on the beach often. Sometimes on the walk Susan would get tired so she would stop and sit cross legged on the soft forest floor or warm sand until she was rested. He would help her up by holding her hand and putting his hand on her waist. On their walks they told each other their secrets, dreams, hurts, and passions.

She told him about her relationship with her parents and what they were like. They were loose and maybe even too permissive. Because of that she did not feel a sense of security and wondered if they cared about her because they put so little effort into raising her.

One day she sat very close to him and smiled so on a whim Eric leaned over and gave her a kiss which lingered for a few seconds.

She was glad that he finally kissed her which meant that their relationship was becoming more serious.

When they walked closely on the beach they would brush against each other as they avoided pieces of driftwood and remnants of campfires on the beach. They wondered who had started the little fires and whether it was a loud group or just two people who were very much in love. He would hold her hand to keep her from falling as they walked through the loose dry sand.

They went out to inexpensive little sushi bars and organic food restaurants often and would order and eat slowly to spend just a little bit of extra time with each other. They always went to restaurants with soft surfaces on the walls and floors so it was not too noisy.

Susan thought about having a fairy tale marriage in which they would always be infatuated with each other. They would never yell at each other and never go to bed without resolving hurt feelings. She started thinking about white picket fences and organic gardens in the backyard.

He would buy her bunches of wildflowers which she would love and put in water as soon as she got home.

They would hold hands as they walked through charming small towns with antique one block long downtowns and stand against each other as they window shopped.

Shopkeepers would look at Eric and Susan and say "You two are a cute couple." They both had thought so but liked having someone notice.

After wearing themselves out while walking through the

historic small town they decided to rest and have dinner at a small French restaurant they came across. They walked in and lingered in a booth and played footsie for some time before ordering. The owner stepped over to their table and told them that he and his lovely wife, Tasha, operated Le Petit Maison. They moved to the United States from France four years ago where he had been a master chef for 20 years and she had been an incredibly talented watercolor artist. The walls were filled with oil paintings, Tasha's watercolors, and photographs of art that is displayed in the precious Louvre. A small artistic replica of the Eiffel tower sat on a small antique table in the corner.

The owner suggested that Eric try a small plate of escargot. The owner told him they were small snails in a butter sauce. Not wanting to appear afraid, he ordered them, ate all of them, but told Susan he was glad he tried them but he would not do so again. As they waited for the next course Susan imagined herself walking with Eric down the Champs - Elysees at sunrise smelling the wonderful aroma of fresh croissants and espresso from the little bistros along the way.

A wonderful feature of this romantic city are the street artists who display their beautiful paintings in outdoor makeshift galleries such as the Montmartre Artist's Market.

Susan and Eric would spend hours pursuing the many outdoor galleries and watching the artists pour their creativity onto an inviting blank canvas. They wandered through the little backstreets dining on small portions of rich French food so as not to make them sluggish as they experienced the little wonders of the large city. As evening drew near they walked back to the boutique hotel and each retired to their room just across the hall from each other.

Every room in the hotel was uniquely designed by a different interior decorator and each one reflected their own creativity and style. Each had soft lighting from ornate fixtures and delicately patterned wallpaper on each wall. The wallpaper in Susan's room was pink and white ordained with tiny pink roses. The pink colored comforter was selected to enhance the room's decor. Susan felt that someone made the room special for her that very night. She curled up in the plush comforter surrounded by small linen cover pillows looking forward to the very next day.

The wall's in Eric's room were filled with oil paintings of Paris purchased by the owner of the hotel to help these passionate artists who do what they love but make little money at it and can barely support themselves.

Some take a 9-5 but plan their next creation during the idle hours of the day. Some waited tables part time which gave them enough money to survive.

The artists would stay at the outdoor gallery until the sun had set and no one could see their works of art.

The artists drifted off to bed so grateful they had the time to do what they loved but unsure of where they would buy lunch tomorrow. Many stayed in underground apartments in the Eiffel Tower district which looked like an 18th century dungeon.

Saturday and Sunday after a small cup of rich coffee the artists would sell their paintings all day long. Susan imagined herself asking an artist about what inspired their work, and then buying a very small painting that could fit in a suitcase.

Susan shared what she had been thinking about with Eric and he said that they could go to Paris later that year. She told Eric that she had to see the Latin Quarter where so many students and professors walked on the wide sidewalks which were perfect for the many young people in that district.

When they finished eating the delicious food they thanked the man and his wife for a wonderful evening and for cooking his steak well done even though the chef felt it ruined it.

When they stepped out the door they noticed how clear the sky was and how visible the stars were which was a fitting conclusion to a wonderful evening.

In front of the restaurant they noticed an older man with a makeshift flower stand that sold single long stemmed red roses with ferns and baby's breath. He bought her one and she just held it to her side as they walked home.

He gently took her hand as they walked close to each other which always delighted her. He had strong hands but held her hand gently as their palms met each other. He was always affectionate which she just loved.

They did go to Paris later that year. Susan anticipated the trip so much that she started packing three weeks before. They boarded the plane and Susan was so excited that she could not sleep at all on the 8 hour flight. Eric drifted off but Susan would wake him up every hour or so to tell him how excited she was. He would stay awake for a while to share her excitement and then go back to sleep. When they landed Susan quickly looked for a cab so they could see the city. They took it to their hotel on the outskirts of town and will always remember the simple roadway sign that just said "Paris". They visited the Louvre and the Mona Lisa which they were mesmerized by. The guards and the railing and the crowds did not deter them from enjoying the painting immensely. They walked the charming streets of the city and purchased small paintings from the street artists. They enjoyed croissants every morning and Eric would eat three but Susan only a half of one.

After they returned from Paris they would go for coffee and brunch often in little out of the way places. She liked being thin so she ate almost nothing.

They remembered he stood very close to her even while they were leading emotional support group meetings and she always leaned ever so slightly towards him. The members of the group were thrilled by their budding romance and would giggle as Eric and Susan looked into each other's bright blue eyes and smiled.

They walked through forests of fruit trees and Eric said she looked so beautiful with the sun rays peeking through the branches and landing on her clear, soft, unblemished, light colored face.

He would enjoy the contrast of tall pine trees to her rather petite figure and would photograph her standing against the forest growth.

The ferns were taller than she was so she could get lost in them and he pictured himself as her knight in shining armor who found her and guided her back to the safe pathway.

He liked her pretty unblemished smooth face, slender figure, and her long blond hair tied in a pony-tail. He loved her sparkling blue eyes which accentuated her naturally pretty face.

They were so much in love and enjoyed being together immensely. They went out to quaint little restaurants and dared each other to try something unusual.

He picked bright
wildflowers of all colors
for her often. He knew
she liked pink roses so he
got up early in the
morning and bought two
dozen as they arrived at
the store and were fresh
and fragrant.

They would hold hands
wherever they went and
look deeply into each
other's blue eyes. He
would give her a light kiss

as he walked her to her house and then he walked to his. He made her rich, flavorful Italian roast coffee and she brewed chamomile tea for him to calm his nerves.

He wore jeans because she felt he looked good in them and she wore cute brightly colored party dresses which he liked seeing her in. She needed to eat a little chocolate every day so he bought small boxes of them every week. They would curl up on the couch and watch romance movies while eating caramel corn.

Neither was afraid to cry at the sappy parts of the show. They did not see any purpose in violence so they avoided movies about war and crime. They insisted on movies

that challenged the mind
and spirit so they avoided
movies that were
simplistic and predictable.
They enjoyed
independent films about
avoiding societal evils and
welcoming characteristics
of humanity.

They were both highly
educated so they often
chose movies that
focused on the academic
significance of the social

sciences, physical sciences, and architecture.

While being entertained by the movie he would kiss her gently and hold her long straight blond hair which she had not cut since he met her. He told her she was beautiful which she never got tired of hearing. She enjoyed the little kisses and hugs that he gave her often and would dress for

him in attractive colorful
clothing.

He bought her flowers that
matched how she dressed.
When she was wearing party
dresses with a colorful pattern
on them he would buy her a
Spring mix of sunflowers,
daisies, lavender, lilies,
daffodils, periwinkle, azalea,
and violet.

 She loved those bright
flowers and would trim them

and put them in a vase immediately to keep them fresh. When she was advocating for our ecology he would pick small bunches of wildflowers to spur her on and inspire her.

He scouted out forests that had a few people on the path so they would be secure but few enough that they could feel alone and experience the cool mist, light winds, and small animals prancing in the meadows. She became mesmerized by small salamanders sitting on rocks who scattered when she bent over to look at them. Eric liked it when she did that because he could see the little girl in her.

She quietly watched the little forest creatures and smiled as they quickly moved away when she approached them and she got so excited when she saw a deer with fawns hiding behind a cluster of trees.

They both wore colorful baseball caps to protect them from the sun because they were both fair skinned.

In the late afternoon on a very long unspoiled beach they built a small fire to stay warm. She leaned against him as their fire turned to coals which were brilliant against the cool misty fog. He gave her a little kiss on the back of her neck and she leaned back towards him.

It was getting chilly and they both were dressed in light cotton clothing which was perfect for their walk but not warm enough for the evening chill so they extinguished the fire and walked home through sand dunes dotted with wildflowers and natural grasses.

On a walk through a pine forest she was delighted to see several baby bunny rabbits hopping through the forest. During their hike they stopped to enjoy a picnic of cheese, muffins, berries, a little chocolate, and several bottles of the clearest spring water they could buy.

The next day they attended a poetry reading held in the corner of an old brick building. Eric had a passion for historical architecture and was delighted with the original brick walls with just enough mortar between the bricks to keep the building from collapsing. He was admiring them when Susan nudged him because the poetry reading was about to begin.

The first poet was a slender man wearing a black t-shirt, canvas shorts, sandals, and bright blue beads.

His poem was about the need for environmental justice which is the premise that the poor should have just as clean an environment as the rich and an extension of that premise is that if we provide clean air and water for the poor we should provide financial security for them as well.

They became members of a nature preservation club which they both enjoyed and felt the members looked deeply at life as Eric and Susan did.

She rented a cute antique home that they hung out in. She had a flair for interior design so she picked out the furniture, drapes, and many, many pillows. The house was full of Tiffany style lamps adorned with a patchwork of brightly colored glass, hand carved wood, antique furniture, and artistic black and white photographs of nature's beauty.

He preferred black and white photos because he felt that color detracted from what the photographer was trying to capture. Each bathroom had a clawfoot bathtub and an antique bench covered with light blue patterned cloth. She had a poster bed complete with a velvet canopy, and a plush bright red antique loveseat.

One quiet afternoon they visited a small town that had a community center and a small museum. There was a dusty sign on the wall which read maximum occupancy 34 which was sufficient for the events that took place there. No one knew how long the center had been there but a historical preservation architect surmised that it was well over a hundred years old. No one really knew who owned the community center and the museum. There was no lock on the door and it did not even have an address, but it was open to everyone.

The small town contained a gentrified warehouse district where local residents had renovated an old brick factory that still looked the same as when it was built in 1884.

During a drive through town, Eric and Susan saw a few people protesting in front of the town's abortion clinic impugning the girl's virtues and condemning those who performed the abortions. They did this in a sensational manner rather than a dignified and loving one.

Although Eric was against abortion, except to save the life and health of the mother, he saw the girls as victims who needed society's assistance so he donated a little money to an organization that helped these girls.

They would often eat at the retro lunch counter in Mr. Walton's pharmacy. He served chocolate milkshakes and little turkey and tomato sandwiches with the crusts cut off. The overhead lighted sign was seventy years old and surrounded by a large number of amber lights.

Many were burnt out but it was still easy to read the sign. Every few weeks a nostalgia buff would photograph the sign and publish the image in a local magazine or blog.

One day as they were walking on an almost deserted foggy beach Eric dropped to one knee on the sand and told Susan he loved her and asked if she would marry him. She gleefully said yes. He reached into the pocket of his windbreaker and removed a one carat, brilliant cut, almost colorless diamond ring and slipped it onto her finger. She slowly folded her left hand to feel it, looked at it, then touched the diamond with the first finger on her right hand and slowly slid her finger off.

Then they romantically kissed and hugged and smiled at each other knowing that they were who they were meant to be.

www.ingramcontent.com/pod-product-compliance
Lightning Source LLC
Chambersburg PA
CBHW070659250726
48662CB00001B/195